PREPARING TO "GO IT ALONE"

Things to Know and Do
Before and After Your Spouse Dies

PREPARING TO "GO IT ALONE"

Things to Know and Do
Before and After Your Spouse Dies

Ruth "Robin" Delaney, CFP, CLU, ChFC

To Doug Van Dyke, my coach, whose encouragement and constant support made this book possible.

About the Author

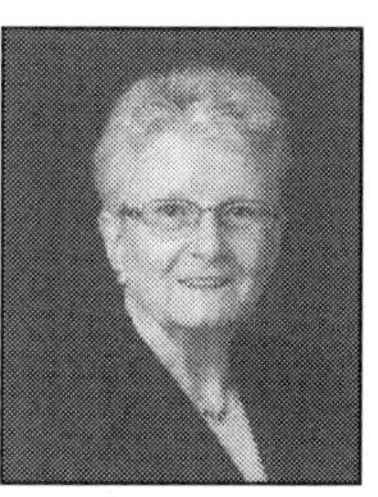

Ruth E. "Robin" Delaney, CFP®, CLU, ChFC, ADPA is a nationally known financial educator, author, speaker and wealth manager based in Tampa, Florida. She has been interviewed in various media, including on FOX TV's WTVT. Her passion is helping both women and men who are on their own, as well as successful families and business owners who are retired or about to retire to experience true financial freedom through a unique process that she developed.

Robin has a passion for lifetime learning. After earning a BA in Mathematics and Economics from Regis College, Robin continued her advanced education by obtaining a MBA in Finance from Hofstra University and an MS in Accounting from Adelphi University. Her relentless pursuit of excellence has led her to obtain additional professional designations, including Certified Financial Planner (CFP), Chartered Life Underwriter (CLU) and Chartered Financial Consultant (ChFC). Robin has also joined the Ed Slott Elite Advisor program and has attained the level of Master Elite Advisor.

Her decades of professional experience, including as a Senior Benefits consultant at one of the Big Four accounting firms, PriceWaterhouseCoopers, equipped her as she launched her own planning and wealth management firm, Greenleaf Financial Strategies,

Inc. She has since merged that firm with Concierge Financial Organization.

As Founder and CEO of an independent financial planning firm, Robin can put her clients' interest first, without pressure to promote products for a financial firm.

As the oldest of eight children, Robin was born to a Navy physician and his wife. As a Pediatric Cardiologist, Robin's father dedicated his life, first to helping heal the children of military personnel, then to serving the children of Long Island, New York.

Because the apple doesn't fall far from the tree, Robin continues the family tradition of helping and serving people, as she guides her clients through their financial lives.

A strong believer in community involvement, Robin has been a board member of A Brighter Community, a not-for-profit preschool and daycare center for at-risk children in the Tampa Bay area since 1998. Robin has served as the past president and board treasurer.

When she is not working, Robin loves spending time with her dog, Mickey, as well as playing golf and taking pictures.

Printed in the United States

First Edition 2017

20 19 18 17 16 5 4 3 2 1

ISBN: 978-0-9991368-0-5

Cover image Shutterstock.com

Edited by Connie Anderson, Words & Deeds, Inc.

Cover and Interior design by Sue Stein

Table of Contents

Introduction

Over the years, I have helped numerous men and women who have lost their spouses. In fact, I helped guide my mother as she navigated a widow's financial landscape. Most women are strong and competent people. However, difficult circumstances can sometimes leave them fragile. Regardless, we all need help and reassurance when coping with grief. While this book was initially intended for women, men sometimes find themselves also needing help in this area. I have, therefore, broadened the scope to include widowers. However, I will refer to all as widows.

While it is always desirable to do advanced planning prior to the loss of your life partner, some of us find ourselves thrust into an unanticipated situation. The emotional aftershock of losing a loved one makes the demands that our financial world imposes on us more difficult.

If you and your spouse have the time to plan ahead, I would suggest that you start with the last chapter first in order to prepare you for the day you are left alone.

Even if you and your spouse had done advanced planning, and you had time to say your goodbye, the reality of death has left you feeling lost. It seems as if you are in a fog. Some have described their disorientation as "trying to walk under water."

Perhaps you were the partner who handled the finances. Now, however, financial matters may feel overwhelming. On the other hand, maybe he/she took care of all the financial details and now it is up to you to handle the affairs of the household. It can feel quite lonely without the other person around to ask for help and financial direction. The intent of this book is to give you guidance and help you through the tumultuous financial aspects of recent widowhood.

You are facing many challenges right now, and you may be emotionally unprepared to handle everything on your own. There is help available, and you simply need to request assistance. My advice is to start with your trusted Financial Advisor.

Remember:

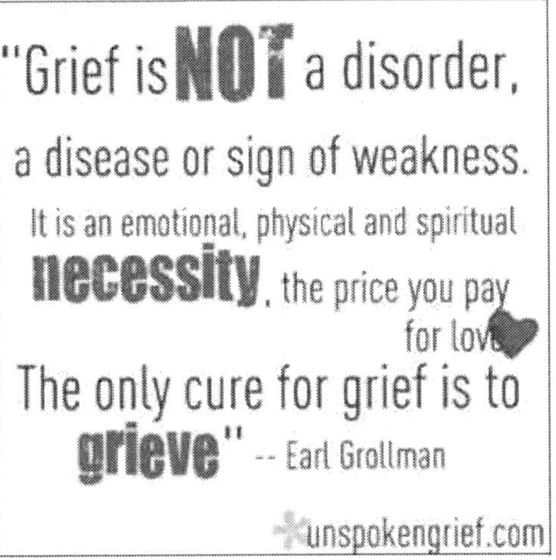

Chapter One

What To Do First

What do I do now?

In 2006, Alan, a strapping man who had just turned fifty, collapsed and died of a massive heart attack while attending Sunday morning Mass with his wife, Karen. Alan and Karen co-owned a business. Alan was a contractor and Karen handled the accounting and billing. Karen was fairly savvy financially. However, because she felt she had to get everything settled "right away" after Alan's passing, she made several costly mistakes. She also started to work while on autopilot instead of thinking strategically. She immediately invested life insurance proceeds. Karen later said, "A friend of mine introduced me to her broker, and I just gave him the money to invest. What a mistake!" The broker proceeded to put her in a series of investments that made no sense for her and her financial situation. Two years later, when she realized what her broker had done, she began to search for a true wealth advisor.

"I wish someone had told me to slow down.
I was so upset when Al died that I just

went into a frenzy. I thought that if I kept busy, the pain of Al's loss would not feel so bad. Instead, I made some bad choices."

Many women like Karen, when faced with the loss of their spouse, feel they must get everything done in a hurry. It is important to realize that you do not have to do everything at once. Many decisions may be made later. More importantly, key decisions should be left to a time when you are not in the initial stages of grief. You will then be able to think more clearly about what is right for you and your family. Do not allow anyone to pressure you into making any major decisions right away. Many widows fall victim to financial predators who take advantage of their vulnerable state. In fact, I recommend that you *do not* make any major life decisions in the year following your spouse's death. If you need help during that time, contact your Financial Advisor and/or your attorney who can help you work through many of these duties. The next few paragraphs detail key actions (or non-actions) to consider after the passing of your loved one.

Death leaves a heartache no one can heal,
love leaves a memory no one can steal.
–From a headstone in Ireland

1. You will need to obtain certified death certificates. Your funeral home director will order these for you. Your Financial Advisor or attorney should be able to help you determine the proper number to order. Then add five (5) more as a cushion for unseen needs.
2. Contact your life insurance agent, or Financial Advisor to help you claim the payment of any death benefits from life insurance policies.

3. Notify your spouse's employer (or former employer, if he/she was retired). A representative of the human resources department at his employer will walk you through the benefits that you are entitled to as his widow. These may include a pension plan, a 401(k) plan, health insurance benefits and group term life insurance. If he was receiving a pension payment, there may be an adjustment made to this benefit due to his death.

   IMPORTANT: DO NOT make any hasty decisions regarding pension, IRA, 401(k), 403(b), 457 or Thrift Savings (TSP) plan assets. Consult a qualified Financial Advisor (preferably an Ed Slott Elite Advisor: find one at www.irahelp.com) to help you navigate the proper resolution of these assets. Hasty or ill-informed decisions may cost you thousands of dollars in taxes that doing careful advanced planning could avoid. I cannot stress that enough. **YOU DO NOT HAVE TO MAKE DECISIONS IMMEDIATELY.** You and your children will generally have until October 31st of the year following your spouse's death to finalize your decisions for these plans.
4. If your spouse was a veteran, contact the Veterans Administration. Prior to contacting the Veterans Administration, collect all the paperwork connected to your spouse's service (i.e., the DD 214 discharge papers).
5. If your spouse was collecting Social Security, contact the Social Security Administration. They will cease his monthly payments and work with you to start or adjust your benefits. Social Security also has a death benefit payment ($255) that you may be entitled to as his widow. If you have dependent children, they may also be eligible for benefits.
6. Contact the attorney who prepared your Wills or Trusts. If you no longer have a relationship with that attorney, your Financial Advisor will be able to recommend one to you. The attorney

will walk you through the larger task of settling your spouse's estate. You have nine (9) months following the death of your spouse to settle the estate. **DO NOT** rush into the estate settlement process and potentially make mistakes that you cannot reverse.

7. Collect all your household bills and ensure that they are paid (i.e., current). You may want to check whether any quarterly tax payments are due. If your spouse paid these online, you may have to locate the website user IDs and passwords for various financial institutions. Later, you will create a budget with your Financial Advisor. (Hint: As a couple, you should share—and then write down each other's passwords, PIN numbers and ID for all computer uses. See Chapter 7: Digital Assets.)

The above information is summarized in the easy to use checklist that appears below.

Checklist of Things to Do First

- ☐ **Contact:**
  - ☐ Attorney
  - ☐ Accountant
  - ☐ Financial Advisor
  - ☐ Life Insurance Agent

- ☐ **Compile the necessary documents:**
  - ☐ Death certificate (10-25 copies)
  - ☐ Marriage certificate
  - ☐ Birth certificates (you, your spouse and any dependent children)
  - ☐ Life insurance policies
  - ☐ Your spouse's Will or Trust

- ☐ Veterans discharge papers
- ☐ Social Security numbers (you, your spouse and any dependent children)
- ☐ Benefit booklets from employer or labor union
- ☐ Complete list of all property and other assets

☐ **Pay the monthly bills:**

- ☐ Gather the bills
- ☐ Locate user IDs and passwords for financial accounts
- ☐ Put together a monthly budget

☐ **Claim and collect benefits owed:**

- ☐ Life insurance
- ☐ Social Security Insurance (SSI) and death benefit, if eligible
- ☐ Social Security benefits for dependent children
- ☐ Veterans death benefits
- ☐ Employee group insurance
- ☐ Union death benefits

Chapter Two

What To Do and Not Do The First Month

Weeks One and Two

After your spouse's funeral and internment, the most important thing is taking care of yourself and your family. Take time to grieve and acknowledge the grief of your family members, especially your children. Unfortunately, there are details that require immediate attention. To help guide you through this process, contact your trusted Financial Advisor, attorney, life insurance agent, and accountant. They will assist you in gathering the important documents outlined in chapter one. They will also help you make important contacts.

Make certain to keep good notes on all your conversations.

As you connect with your professional advisors, you may want to enlist the help of a trusted friend or family member to serve as a second pair of eyes and ears. They may help you by taking notes and remembering the important details of conversations. During this time of your extreme grief, a second perspective from this friend or family member may help you sort through the questions you will face, and then enable you to make better decisions.

In 2003 my father passed away leaving my mother to execute the plans they had put in place years before his passing. She had raised eight children and coordinated the moves from station to station every two years during my father's 26-year career in the US Navy. She was a force to be reckoned with when it came to organization and logistics. After 56 years of marriage, this strong, able woman, who handled all the family finances, was devastated and confused. Fortunately, she had her daughter to walk her through the complex, as well as the mundane, tasks of settling his affairs and rearranging her own. This second set of eyes and ears helped her to cope and eventually to make better decisions. Do not underestimate the power of grief to cloud your thinking.

For your immediate financial needs, such as funeral or burial expenses, review your life insurance policies or any pre-arrangement details. Your life insurance agent or Financial Advisor may be quite helpful with this task. Also, ask your Financial Advisor to help you set aside six months of living expenses from the funds you will receive from life insurance or benefits payments. If your spouse was the primary wage earner, this may be very helpful as you put your life back together.

Finally, you will want to ask your funeral director for 10–25 copies of your spouse's death certificate in preparation for the tasks ahead.

Weeks Three and Four

Budgeting

You have attended to your immediate needs in weeks one and

two. Now it is time to meet with your Financial Advisor to begin putting your life back together. Collectively you can look at your finances and make decisions appropriate to your new situation. This will include creating a budget to determine your income needs.

Analyze where your money comes from, and where it goes each month. If you need more money to cover your monthly expenses, look at your portfolio with your Financial Advisor to create a "paycheck" to provide what you need. If your spouse had handled all the family finances, then this will be a learning experience for you. A budget worksheet is included in the Appendix to help guide you in this effort. This will be useful even if you are experienced at budgeting.

Regarding the need for income to cover your monthly expenses, you and your advisor should discuss any changes to your portfolio considering your changed circumstances.

Estate Settlement

With the help of your Financial Advisor, compile a list of all your assets, including your home. This will be necessary when you meet with your attorney to settle your spouse's estate. If you are not the executor/executrix (or personal representative) named in your spouse's Will, have your Financial Advisor contact the person named in the Will, as well as your attorney. These professionals will work together for a smooth transition. If you do not have an attorney, your advisor may be able to recommend one.

Estate settlement can take as little as few months to as much as several years, depending upon the complexity of your financial situation and disposition of your assets. Your attorney can give you a good idea of the anticipated period. For most estates, this time frame is only a few months.

Take all the time you need to heal emotionally. Moving on doesn't take a day. It takes a lot of little steps to be able to break free of your broken self.

Retirement Benefits

This area requires a great deal of attention to detail. Mistakes in this area could cost you thousands of dollars in taxes. If your Financial Advisor is not an expert in this area, you may want to consider searching for an Ed Slott Elite Advisor in your area through the www.irahelp.com website. You have until October 31st of the year following your spouse's death to move these funds. In other words, you have time to settle these accounts in the correct way. **Do not let anyone rush you into making decisions.** Chapter Five contains more detail on this topic.

Questions:

1. Do you have a team of trusted advisors to help you?
   Yes No

2. Can a friend or family member accompany you to take notes?
   Yes No

3. If you are meeting with a new advisor, have you vetted him or her through the appropriate regulatory authorities?
   Yes No

Regulatory and Background Checks:

1. www.FINRA.org (broker check or investment advisor check).
2. www.SEC.org.
3. Check your State division of insurance or securities.

Chapter Three

Important Actions and Decisions During The First Year

This first year will be a time of transition for you. You will experience many "firsts," like birthdays, holidays and other special events to attend without your partner. Let family and friends help you through these times. Support groups and bereavement counseling have helped many men and women cope with their loss. You can locate a local group through www.griefshare.org. There are also other sites on the internet where you can connect with others who are coping with loss.

All the tasks you started in the first month will be ongoing throughout much of the first year. You will be working to shore up your finances so they see you through the remainder of your life. If your spouse's estate is large or complex, you may still be settling the estate with your attorney. Your accountant, attorney and Financial Advisor should all work together to help you organize and work through this process.

Jen lost her beloved Tim to a sudden heart attack. They knew that Tim had heart disease, but his passing was still shocking, nonetheless. When Jen notified one of Ken's retirement account providers of his passing, they sent out an aggressive young man who attempted to pressure Jen into an expensive annuity. She didn't feel right about it and asked a family friend for advice. That friend referred Jen to me.

We talked about the plans she and Tim had made and what she wanted to do with the money that he left her. We discussed their children and the legacy that she and Tim had planned to leave for them. We made some modifications to the plans they had made and rearranged her investments to suit Jen's new circumstances. We then met with her attorney to prepare a new Will.

Like Jen, this is the time to meet with your attorney and your Financial Advisor to create a new estate plan, as well as to draft a new Will or Trust for yourself. Your Financial Advisor will meet with you to make any necessary changes to your beneficiary designations. He or she should make certain that the title on all your accounts are correct and in agreement with your new estate plan.

After you have completed your new estate planning documents, sit down with your family to discuss your financial situation, and you may want to invite your Financial Advisor to this meeting. Part of the discussion should cover your wishes in the event of your serious illness or death.

Then, begin planning for taxes with your accountant and Financial Advisor. Your tax situation will change now that you are widowed. You will find more about this in Chapter Six.

Depending upon how your home is owned, you may need to retitle your homestead. Your attorney can assist you with this and help you determine if you are entitled to a widow's deduction for property taxes. This will depend on the laws of your state and local taxing authority. You may even consider selling your home and moving to a smaller place. Consider this decision carefully.

Making large financial decisions and moves in the first year may be hazardous to your financial health. *Consult your advisors* before making any drastic changes in the first year. These advisors should include your professional advisors, as well as your family and close friends. If family is pressuring you to make decisions that you feel are not in your best interest, let the advisors play the "bad guy" with your family. You do not have to face them alone.

Only in darkness can you see the stars.
–Martin Luther King Jr.

Questions:

1. Are you being pressured to make a financial or life decision?
   Yes No

2. Are you sharing this pressure with your advisory team?
   Yes No

Chapter Four

Understanding Social Security Benefits

When a spouse dies, the survivor can apply for survivor benefits as early as age 60 (50 if you are disabled). If your spouse was receiving benefits when he/she died, the survivor benefit will equal 100% of your spouse's benefit. However, it will be subject to the actuarial reduction if you apply before you have reached your full retirement age.

Age To Receive Full Social Security Benefits (Called "full retirement age" or "normal retirement age.")	
Year of Birth	**Full Retirement Age**
1937 or earlier	65
1938	65 and 2 months
1939	65 and 4 months
1940	65 and 6 months
1941	65 and 8 months

Year of Birth	Full Retirement Age
1942	65 and 10 months
1943–1954	66
1955	66 and 2 months
1956	66 and 4 months
1957	66 and 6 months
1958	66 and 8 months
1959	66 and 10 months
1960	67
*If you were born on January 1st of any year, you should refer to the previous year. (If you were born on the 1st of the month, SSA will figure your benefit (and your full retirement age) as if your birthday was in the previous month.)	

Source: www.ssa.gov

The actuarial reduction is approximately 8% for each year you take Social Security benefits early, and increased by 8% for every year that you delay your benefits beyond your Full Retirement Age (FRA). If your own benefit is the higher of the two, you may want to receive that amount, but you cannot receive both.

If you were both receiving Social Security when your spouse dies, his/her benefit will stop. You can then switch over to his/her benefit, if it is higher. Three things to note about this are:

1. Your survivor benefit would equal your deceased spouse's actual benefit, not the Full Retirement Benefit. If he/she waited until age 70 to apply, your survivor benefit would be higher. If applied for earlier, your survivor benefit would be less.
2. When one spouse dies, one of the benefits will stop. If your benefit was higher, that will be the one you will keep. Either way you will need to plan for this loss of income on one of the benefits. Since most surviving spouses need at least two-thirds

of the income they were receiving as a couple, life insurance or other liquid assets may be needed to fill the gap.

3. If you remarry after being widowed, you will not be eligible for a survivor benefit—unless you are age 60 or older when you remarry (50 if you are disabled).

Questions:

1. Do you have minor children?

   Yes No

2. Do you plan to remarry?

   Yes No

Chapter Five

Accessing Retirement Benefits

This is an area where small omissions can have large consequences. Whenever one's life circumstances change, a review of your beneficiary designations on all your retirement plans is critical.

When working for a large pension plan in New York City, I came across this situation:

> Dr. Brown unexpectedly died in his early fifties. He had been married to his second wife for several years, having divorced his first wife in a very acrimonious and public divorce. He managed to change his Will to leave his estate to the new Mrs. Brown. However, he forgot to change the beneficiary designation on his substantial pension plan benefits. When it was discovered that the first Mrs. Brown was the named beneficiary on the plan, the new Mrs. Brown sued.
>
> Under Federal law a spouse is entitled to half of the pension benefits of a spouse. An employee can name anyone else to inherit the other half, but unless the spouse waives his/her rights in writing to their rightful half, they cannot name a non-spouse as beneficiary of the entire amount. Wills do not govern the

distribution of retirement plan benefits, beneficiary designations do. Therefore, the judge awarded half of the pension plan benefits to the second Mrs. Brown as the legal spouse of Dr. Brown, and half to the first Mrs. Brown as the named beneficiary. This was not what Dr. Brown intended, as he had made a fair settlement with the first Mrs. Brown in their divorce.

It is so important that you review your beneficiary designations on your retirement plans, insurance and annuity policies on a regular basis.

Now, your spouse may have accumulated many retirement benefits during his/her working life. Each broad type is described below with some of the decisions that you will want to consider for your circumstances.

What we have once enjoyed, we can never lose.
All that we love deeply becomes part of us."
–Helen Keller

IRA Accounts

Substantial assets may have accumulated in your spouse's 401(k), 403(b) or a Governmental 457(b) plan. At some point, due to retirement or changes in employment, he/she may have rolled these accounts into an IRA. If you are the sole beneficiary of these accounts, you will have four options for handling the treatment of these accounts.

Option #1 – You may cash in the accounts and pay income taxes on the proceeds. If you choose this option, you may wish to have the company withhold Federal and State taxes so that you are not "caught short" at tax time. You will want to think carefully before choosing this option, particularly if the account balances are large, as the tax burden will greatly reduce the cash amount you will receive. Taking the balance over a period of years will, in most instances, reduce your overall tax burden.

Option #2 – You may elect to treat the account as your own, leaving it invested where it is. You would choose this option if moving the account elsewhere would mean you lose access to certain investments in that account that you wish to keep. You essentially pretend that the account was yours all along, and follow the rules for distributions (required minimum distributions, etc.) as though the account was your own. If you choose this option, either consciously or by default (i.e., inaction on your part), you may not later choose to be treated as a beneficiary (Option #4).

Option #3 – You may elect to roll over the account to your own IRA. In this instance, the account is treated as though it was your IRA account all along. If you are over the age of 59½, this may be a good option for you as you are beyond the 10% penalty phase for early distributions. You would name your own beneficiaries, and when you reach age 70½, you would begin taking your required minimum distributions. This strategy works well if you were younger than your deceased spouse. If he/she was already over 70½ and taking required minimum distributions, you would be able to stop those distributions until you reach 70½.

NOTE: Once you choose this option, you may not later opt for the inherited IRA in Option #4.

If you are older than your deceased spouse, or are under age 59½, you may want to consider Option #4.

Option #4 – You may elect to take the account as an Inherited IRA. The account will have a special title, such as ***John Spouse (deceased mm/dd/yyyy) IRA FBO Jane Spouse.*** You might choose this option if you think you may need to take distributions from the account—and you are under the age of 59½. Distributions from an inherited IRA are not subject to the 10% early distribution penalty. You might also consider this option if you are older than your deceased spouse, and you wish to delay required minimum distributions until he/she would have been 70½.

However, you are not required to take the minimum distributions until your deceased spouse would have reached 70½.

Many younger spouses choose an inherited IRA until they reach age 59½, at which point they choose a spousal rollover (Option #3), thereby delaying the required minimum distributions until they reach 70½.

As you can see, this area is complex, and we have just scratched the surface. There is the potential to create large and unwanted tax consequences. Sometimes difficult choices must be made regarding timing, and you will want an experienced, competent Financial Advisor to guide you through the decision-making process.

401(k), 403(b), Governmental 457(b) and Thrift Savings Accounts

These plans can be rolled over to an IRA, either in your own name or as an inherited IRA. The same choices as outlined above would apply. Review these options with your Financial Advisor to choose the options that are best suited to your situation.

You and your Financial Advisor will want to find out and take into consideration these two things in your planning.

1. If your spouse has a substantial amount of company stock in his 401(k) plan or ESOP, some special tax treatments may be

available to you. Your Financial Advisor or accountant should know how to handle the "net unrealized appreciation" in the stock holdings. Because it's complex—**do not attempt to navigate this area on your own.** Even if you have experience in this area, the emotional stress you are under will make it easy to make a mistake and create an unwanted tax bill.

2. Ask the plan administrator of the 401(k) if there are any after-tax contributions (i.e., your spouse did not get a tax deduction at the time he/she made the contributions to the plan) in the account. New rules will allow you to roll these contributions to a Roth IRA, if the rollover is handled properly.

Pension Plans

Your spouse may already be receiving payments from his/her company/government/union pension plan if he/she has retired. This benefit may be reduced depending on the option that he/she chose at retirement. The plan administrator and your Financial Advisor will guide you through this process.

If your spouse was not yet retired, you may have the choice of a lump sum settlement of his retirement benefit, or a stream of payments. You will want to consult with your Financial Advisor, the plan administrator and your accountant to choose the option that is right for your circumstances.

Questions:

1. Do you know what retirement benefits your spouse had?
   Yes No

2. Do you know who the beneficiaries are for these benefits?
   Yes No

Chapter Six

Knowing What Taxes You'll Pay

Income Taxes

In the year following your spouse's death, many widows and widowers are surprised when they file their first income tax return as a single person to find that they are in a higher tax bracket than when they were filing as a married couple. This is known as the "widow's penalty." If you have dependent children, you will be able to put this off for several years, as you will be able to file as a qualifying widow and use the joint tax rates. However, most widows are retired or are elderly and collecting Social Security benefits.

Single taxpayers move up in the tax brackets more quickly than married taxpayers. If you find that your income after your spouse's death is the same or just slightly smaller than when he/she was alive, you may end up in a higher tax bracket because of this phenomenon. If you and your spouse were high-income earners, some of the deductions that you could take advantage of as a married couple may disappear for you now as a single tax payer.

Government Benefits

Lower middle-income widows, who are receiving Social Security payments, may find that their Social Security benefit may now be partially taxable. Prior to your spouse's death, if your "combined income" was less than $44,000, your Social Security benefits may not have been taxed. If your "combined income" in the year after your spouse's death does not fall below $25,000, *up to 85% of your Social Security benefit may now be taxed.* For higher-income earners, this increase in taxation may not be as much, as you were already paying tax on 85% of your Social Security benefits.

You may also be surprised by the Medicare "stealth" tax, if you are a higher-income earner. Medicare Part B premiums increase for married couples earning more than $170,000, but will also increase for single payers earning just $85,000 or more.

You will want to work with your Financial Advisor and your accountant to implement some planning strategies to offset some of these unwanted tax consequences. You will especially want to work with your accountant to make certain that you do not under-withhold for taxes in that first year after your spouse's passing.

Chapter Seven

Handling Your Spouse's Digital Assets

These days, even more people who are elderly have digital assets. What are digital assets? In short, *any* accounts or sites you own or use online. What grandparent does not have a Facebook account? These digital assets make us increasingly vulnerable to identity theft. It is therefore extremely important to manage your spouse's digital assets after death.

The accounts you need to be concerned about are:

- Email
- Online banking/bill paying
- Online brokerage
- PayPal
- eBay
- Facebook
- LinkedIn
- Twitter

- Photo/video sharing accounts (i.e., Instagram, Flickr, YouTube, etc.)
- Personal websites
- Blogs
- Online backup sites (i.e., Carbonite, Mozy, etc.)

This list is by no means exhaustive as new services are introduced every day. Digital assets and social media is a new area and many of the sites have different policies for removing accounts from the Web. These sites contain sensitive personal information and financial data that could pose privacy concerns if left unattended indefinitely.

If you have not discussed what you would like to happen to your accounts after you are gone, and how your loved ones can access your accounts, here are a few guidelines that you can follow:

Facebook

Facebook has two options for what to do with a deceased family member's account.

1. **Memorializing a profile.** This feature allows the account to be viewed but not edited (except for a legacy contact allowed to make one final post, usually regarding funeral arrangements, etc.).
2. **Terminating an account.** You can deactivate a profile by completing a "Special Request For Deceased Person's Account." It will be necessary to prove your relationship as well as providing a copy of the death certificate, birth certificate or proof of authority for the person handling the deactivation.

LinkedIn

There are two ways to terminate a LinkedIn account.

1. **Password known.** If you have the password, you can just follow LinkedIn's instructions to simply close the account.
2. **Password unknown.** If you do not know the password, and you are an immediate family member, extended family member or non-family member (friend, co-worker, classmate), you may follow the "Process To Terminate An Account" on LinkedIn. You will have to provide information about the deceased and your relationship to the deceased.

Preparation Before Death

Make a List of Your Digital Assets and Accounts

You may want to create a list of your digital assets and accounts by category to help organize your thoughts and ease the process. The categories should include:

- **Hardware:** Include computers, hard drives, back-up drives, flash drives, iPods, cell phones, cameras, etc. You will want to make a list of these items, what is on them, and where they are stored.
- **Software**: Tax preparation software, Quicken, QuickBooks and past tax returns are important. In addition, include Word or Excel documents that might be important.
- **Social Media and Online Presence:** Facebook, Twitter, LinkedIn, Flickr, YouTube, your own website, your blog, online backup sites on which you store photos, documents or other important digital files.

Select a Successor

If you and your spouse have not already discussed whom you would want to access your computer, your email, and your online accounts in your absence, think about whom you would want to assume this task. This person must have good computer knowledge. A younger family member with good computer skills might be a good choice. You will want to talk to this person in advance to let them know of your plans.

Provide Access

You will want to create a list of each account or asset and list the user name, password, PIN numbers, and the sites domain name. You must keep this list updated and secure. Do not keep this list lying around in a desk drawer. You may want to consider a safe deposit box or a home safe. Tell your successor where the list is and how to access it. If you keep it on your computer or "in the cloud," make sure the file is password protected.

The person you name as your successor will need death certificates to close your accounts. Consider naming this person as a co-trustee or co-executor with responsibilities that are limited to this area in order to give them legal authority to act for you.

The only people who think there's a time limit for grief, have never lost a piece of their heart. Take all the time you need.

Provide Instructions

Write down a set of instructions that may be kept with your Will or Trust for your successor. Include those accounts (such as Facebook or your blog) that you would like to be maintained in order to memorialize you after you are gone. You can configure your email to send an auto-response to notify the sender of the death and where to forward information.

You will want to include instructions for saving information, such as photos or videos before sites that are no longer needed are closed. Be as detailed as you can in your instructions. Have your successor check with the attorney or accountant about any data they may need for your estate tax returns prior to closing sites.

Questions:

1. Do you or your spouse have a Facebook, LinkedIn or other social media account?

   Yes No

2. Do you or your spouse do your banking online?

   Yes No

3. Do you or your spouse pay bills online?

   Yes No

4. Do you store your pictures and videos online?

   Yes No

Chapter Eight

Advanced Planning

"All good men and women must take responsibility to create legacies that will take the next generation to a level we could only imagine.
–Jim Rohn

Most of us do not want to deal with the topic of death, and certainly not our own. However, it is something that every couple, no matter their age, should discuss. People of all ages die from accidents, illnesses and other tragedies—not just the older generation. We can leave our loved ones better prepared to face life without us if we discuss it with them, and then take some preliminary actions to smooth the way for those left behind. What if you are the one left behind? Wouldn't you want the transition to living without your partner to be as smooth as possible? So why not do a little planning now? We never know when we must face the inevitable.

Carl (85) and Amy (62) were happily married for 35 years. After their anniversary dinner they were headed home when a drunk driver T-boned their car killing Amy instantly. Carl was heartbroken and confused. They had always planned on Amy taking care of Carl in his final years. Now he was left alone without his soulmate and recordkeeper. Amy had always taken care of their finances as they had anticipated that she would be the one left. Carl was out of his element. Fortunately, they had talked out their plans and we had everything in place for a smooth transition for Carl.

Isn't it strange how life sometimes throws us curveballs.

In the following sections, you will find an outline of some basic steps to take to help ease the transition. Set aside some time to talk about what you would want in the event of your death. You will need to consider end-of-life decisions, funeral arrangements, care of any dependent children, as well as income for the surviving spouse. If you have accumulated substantial wealth, consider how you want that wealth distributed. After you and your spouse have discussed these topics, the next step is to put your plans into action.

Dependent Children

- Discuss any arrangements for guardianship of minor children with your intended guardians to be certain they are willing to accept this responsibility should the need arise.
- For minor children or children with special needs, talk to your attorney and Financial Advisor about establishing the appropriate financial and legal arrangements for their care after you are gone.

Create a Written Plan

- Meet with your Financial Advisor to get your plan in writing and begin the process of putting it in place. Your Advisor should coordinate this process to ensure that everything that is drafted matches your plan. He or she will put together a comprehensive list of your assets and the titling of those assets for the attorney.

- Bring your financial plan to the attorney or have your Financial Advisor send it to him/her in advance of your visit.
- If during the planning process, you realize that there are not enough assets to sustain the remaining family members for an appropriate period, then apply for life insurance to help fill this gap. For a relatively small investment, insurance proceeds can provide an immediate fund, larger than you could save in a short period to help your family cope with the loss of your income or services.
- If you are in your 50's or 60's, and you have accumulated a fair number of assets that you wish to pass on to your heirs, consider purchasing some type of long-term care plan. There are several ways that you can protect your assets in the event you or your spouse requires care for an extended period, whether it is home health care, assisted living or skilled nursing care. You do not want the surviving spouse to have to carry on with a reduced lifestyle because of the other partner's accident or chronic illness.

Estate Settlement

- You will first need a Will or a Trust, depending on the type of assets that you own. If you do not have an estate plan or elder law attorney, your Financial Advisor may recommend one. The attorney will put together a comprehensive package of documents to handle the settlement of your estate. These documents should at least also include a Living Will and a Durable Power of Attorney, along with your Will and/or Trust. Other documents may be needed based on your situation.

- If your spouse will not be your personal representative for your estate, talk to whomever you wish to fill this role to be certain that he or she is willing and able to assume this responsibility. Also, consider having co-representatives or an alternate selected in case the first person cannot serve when needed.
- Have your Advisor review all beneficiary designations for your insurance and retirement plans to ensure that they conform to your wishes.
- Discuss your wishes regarding your digital assets. Make a list of sites that contain personal information or actual assets. You will want to consider PayPal, eBay, personal business, photo sharing and social networking sites, etc. Make these wishes known to your attorney and your Financial Advisor so that they may be incorporated into your estate planning.

Funeral Arrangements

If you or your spouse have special wishes regarding the handling of his/her remains, you should discuss it. You may want to look into pre-planning your funeral arrangements if you are both retired or if there are health issues.

Once you have your plans in place, as a couple you should talk to your family, if your children are old enough, and broadly explain your plan to them. Let everyone know whom your advisors are and how to get in touch with them in the event that they need to put your plans into action.

You may wish to put together a binder with important information for your family. You will want to keep this binder in a safe and secure place. This binder could include the following:

1. A list of your advisors and their contact information.
2. A copy of your Will or Trust, if you are not housing it with your attorney.

3. Copies of any funeral arrangements you may have made in advance.
4. Any special instructions for your funeral arrangements that you would like your loved ones to follow.
5. A list of your passwords to all of your online accounts.
6. Instructions of how to locate important documents that your family may need such as:
   a. Birth certificates
   b. Military discharge papers
   c. Deeds to property
   d. Car titles (unless your state keeps them digitally), etc.
7. Love letters you've written to your family members to be opened after you are gone.

Today is the right day to begin planning and talking to family members. It is never too soon to prepare, as we never know what life will bring.

Questions:

1. Do you have a Will or a Trust?
   Yes No
2. Do you know where all your important papers are stored?
   Yes No
3. If you have minor children, have you thought about who you want to take care of them if you are not there?
   Yes No
4. Have you each talked about what you want if you are the first to go?
   Yes No

I wish you all the best on your life's journey. Sometimes life is difficult. Sometimes life, despite its hurdles, is wonderful. Perhaps, my friend, it is ours to choose. Be well.

–Robin

Appendix

Budget Worksheet

An annual budget shows where your money comes from and how you spend it for both necessary and discretionary expenses. Complete the worksheet below by recording the average monthly expense in the left-hand column and then fill in the annual amount. This will give you a snapshot of how your money flows. Try to complete this before you see your Financial Advisor and he/she will help you to fine-tune it.

Income	Average Month ($)	Annual ($)
Job 1 (take-home pay)		
Job 2 (take-home pay)		
Interest		
Dividends and Capital Gains		
Social Security		
Income from Business or Partnership		
Sale of an Investment or other asset		
Life Insurance Proceeds		
Rental Income		
Other:		
Total Income	$	$

Necessary Expenses	Average Month ($)	Annual ($)
Mortgage or Rent		
Home Maintenance		
Groceries		
Utilities and Phone/Internet		
Transportation costs, gasoline and upkeep		
Clothing and cleaning		
Personal and self-care		
Medical, Dental and other health care		
Debt or loan repayment		
Insurance: home and property		
Insurance: car		
Insurance: life		
Insurance: disability		
Insurance: long-term care		
Real Estate Taxes		
Taxes: quarterly estimated taxes		
Other:		
Other:		
Total Necessary Expenses	$	$

Discretionary Expenses	Average Month ($)	Annual ($)
Vacation and leisure travel		
Dining out		
Recreation		
Entertainment		
Gifts: charitable		
Gifts: family and friends		
Home Furnishings		

Discretionary Expenses	Average Month ($)	Annual ($)
Savings: emergency fund		
Savings: retirement		
Savings: college		
Investments		
Family support		
Children or grandchildren		
Hobbies		
Subscriptions and dues		
Pet care		
Memberships		
Other: ________________		
Total Discretionary Expenses	$	$

Annual Summary	
Total Income	$
Subtract **Total Necessary Expenses**	−$
Subtract **Total Discretionary Expenses**	−$
Circle one **Excess or Shortage**	$

About Ed Slott

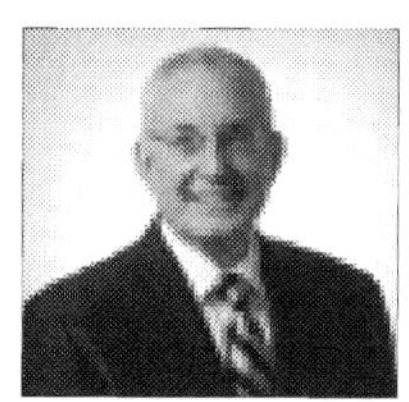

Ed Slott was named *"The Best" source for IRA advice* by the *Wall Street Journal.*

He is a nationally recognized professional speaker and has starred in several nationally aired public television specials including the most recent, *Ed Slott's Retirement Road Map* (2017).

Slott created the *Ed Slott's Elite IRA Advisor Group*™, which was developed specifically to help financial professionals earn recognition as leaders in the IRA marketplace. This exclusive organization of financial advisors is dedicated to being leaders in the IRA industry. Ed Slott's Elite IRA Advisors are equipped with up-to-date tools and resources to help their clients.

Mr. Slott is an accomplished author of many financial and retirement-focused books including most recently *Ed Slott's Retirement Decisions Guide: 2017 Edition* (IRAHelp, 2017), and *Fund Your Future: A Tax-Smart Savings Plan in Your 20s and 30s* (IRAHelp, 2015). Slott also publishes *Ed Slott's IRA Advisor,* a monthly IRA newsletter. He is a personal finance columnist for numerous financial publications.

As a thought leader in the retirement industry, Slott is often quoted in the *New York Times, Wall Street Journal, Forbes, Money, Kiplinger's, USA Today, Investment News* and a host of additional national magazines and financial publications. He has appeared on numerous national television and radio programs. Mr. Slott is also a consultant to financial information websites.

For more information:

Website: www.irahelp.com
Email: info@irahelp.com
Twitter: @theslottreport
Facebook: AmericasIRAExperts
LinkedIn: Ed Slott & Company
YouTube: EdSlottandCompanyIRA

Made in the USA
Columbia, SC
12 September 2017